WAITING

· · ·

568 THOUGHTS

WHILE WAITING FOR A HEART TRANSPLANT

Kate O'Boyle

Greg & Edwina -

#335

I hope everyone can experience the feeling of making a difference.

Thank you for all you have done for humanity.

you & me

BEST

Kate

Printed in the United States of America
First Printing, 2019

ISBN: 978-1-947703-05-6

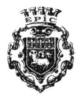

E.P.I.C. Publishing Services, LLC
P.O. Box 182
Hadlyme, CT 06439

BOOK DESIGN BY RUSSELL C. SHADDOX

ACKNOWLEDGMENTS

I would be remiss if I did not thank the people and institutions that were an integral part of my journey. The following have my undying gratitude.

- Donor and Donor Family
- Charlene Riling, who is my rock, caregiver, biggest cheerleader, and my world
- The Franko Family
- The Slivka Family
- The O'Boyle Family
- The Riling Family
- Brian Armstrong
- Sheila Osko whose connection to Brigham and Women's Hospital, started me on my medical and healing journey
- Dr. Lynne Warner Stevenson, MD
- The great doctors and nurses at Brigham and Women's Hospital in Boston, MA
- LVAD Clinic Team at Brigham and Women's Hospital
- The Heart Transplant Team at Brigham and Women's Hospital
- Dr. Carolyn Kosack, MD
- St. Francis Hospital in Hartford, CT
- Donate Life CT/New England/America
- Rebecca Barton LPC
- Lincoln Financial Group, for living up to its mission and core values
- My relatives, friends, and acquaintances, who provided me with endless emotional and spiritual support

SPECIAL ACKNOWLEDGMENTS

- John W. and Grace H. O'Boyle – my parents, who raised a strong woman.
- Sean Franko (below left) 1976 – 2011; my nephew, a heart transplant recipient, and a source of inspiration. I love you!
- Dennis Franko, Jr. (below right) 1975 – 2013; my nephew who left us far too soon but is always with me. I love you!

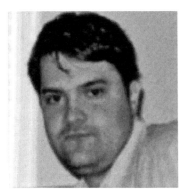 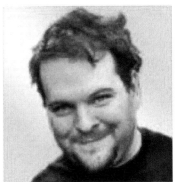

AUTHOR'S NOTE

Pre-Transplant

Listed below are the activities and actions that were important to me during this stage of my journey:

- Meditating, a positive attitude, writing, and helping others were keys to my being. While I was helping others, I was helping myself. It kept my mind off things and allowed me to concentrate on others. Don't get me wrong, I still had moments when fear and anger would enter the picture, but I found that in setting some time aside for these feelings and working through them, it made me stronger.
- Reading was important. I read self-help and spirituality books, then practiced the lessons learned.
- Continuing to live my life and not becoming a prisoner to my condition was important to me. I did not want to be Kate, the cardiac patient. I wanted to be Kate, who just so happens to have a cardiac condition.
- A sense of humor helped me through these pre-transplant days. When I was able to laugh at myself and my predicament, I was bringing a sense of relief not only to myself but to others. It lightened the situation and gave friends and family the opportunity to be themselves and not have to worry about what to say to me while I was dealing with a critical illness.
- Exercise, exercise, exercise, was my mantra. I formulated my own work out routines and made a schedule for myself. I would work out 5 days per week and stick to that routine. As a matter of fact, my phone call for transplant came when I was at the gym and on the treadmill. This was truly fitting.

Post-Transplant

Post-transplant is a continuation of my pre-transplant life, with gratitude being the apex. Gratitude to the donor, donor family, and the donor heart are constants in my life. Not a day goes by that I don't reflect on how this has changed my world forever. I journal and give thanks daily for my new life.

Listed below are personal changes that I have noted:

- I feel things more deeply. It is not that I didn't before, but there is a noticeable difference.
- My emotions can be intense.
- I have a deeper respect for **all** people.
- I empathize with others who have chronic illness. The first 6 months following my transplant, I had prednisone induced diabetes, tremors, and needed to take daily injections: insulin (6 months) and fondaparinux for blood clots (3 months).
- I am very sensitive to the plight of others.
- Injustices in the world affect me. I get emotional seeing how people are being treated and how they treat each other.
- The need to give back is very strong.
- The notion that I am here for a reason comes to me often. Drilling down to what that reason is, sends me on an introspective journey.
- The nighttime sky and nature are important to me.
- Peanut butter, walnuts, and spicy foods are irresistible.

Finally, there are times when I feel I am losing my harmony with the universe. I get distracted by the negative in the world and lose sight of all that is good. I start to spend too much time wondering why bad things happen, instead of wondering about the good around me and ways to spread that joy. When this happens, I go back to what brought that harmony: meditating, reading, music, writing, exercising, helping others, and resisting the negativity. I realize now that I am a warrior, always on guard against the invaders of my personal and social-emotional space. Every day is a battle and thus far, I am happy to report, I am holding my own in the fight.

INTRODUCTION

The years 2008–2014 were life altering. Having been diagnosed with heart failure in March of 2008 and having it confirmed in April with talk of heart transplant, was beyond my comprehension. The many thoughts that ran through my mind were overwhelming.

What follows here are 568 thoughts I recorded over the course of 6 years. It chronicles the ups and downs of my healing journey, dealing with loss, and searching for a new purpose in life. The only change I have made to my thoughts is spelling. The sentence structure or lack thereof, remains the same.

If you have had or are experiencing a major life change, I hope these thoughts are ones you can take with you while you make sense of the path which lies ahead.

2008

1

March 17th came with a vengeance
and remains ...

2

Life Vest takes on a new meaning ...
it truly is a "life" vest ...

3

You over focus; that's what you try not
to do ...

4

We are here for more blood ... Really?

5

Black and blue are my favorite colors ...

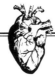

6

I cannot believe this ...
this is surreal ... I wish I could wake up
and it would all be over!

7

I get my moments, but I refuse
to give in ...

8

Friends, who knew I had so many ...

9

Be good to everyone you meet ...
they deserve it, you deserve it ...

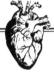

10

People do care ...

11

People will help,
all you need to do is ask ...

12

I am fortunate I am loved!

13

How do you go from everything
to nothing?

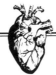

14

My life vest on, my anxiety high
but I am happy to be going home ...

15

Charlene is my life, my world,
my refuge, and my comfort!

16

I want her to know everything
will be all right ... I want her to tell me
everything will be all right ...

17

This is not the program I had in mind!

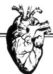

18

I think of school, but I should
be thinking of myself ...

19

Hawks are interesting creatures …
now I watch him like a hawk!

20

Failing Heart-Failing School – ironic …
but not for long!

21

This is a bad April's Fool joke,
and I don't get it!

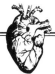

22

I have waited 2 weeks, let's go
and see what the future holds ...

23

Divine interventions come
in the most mysterious of ways ...

24

Thank You God!

25

What do I do next?

26

There are many trade-offs when you
are a highly trained professional ...

27

I am going through my stuff ...
shred the insignificant ...

28

Shredding makes you review
your entire life up until this point!
What an exercise!

29

How fortunate am I!

30

I pray and thank God everyday ...

31

Is a heart transplant inevitable I ask ... ?
The doctor responds she wouldn't use
those words, she would use likely ...

32

I like having dreams with mom in
them, it's like I have her with me ...

33

I am still figuring out
what I want to do ...

34

It's funny how things go around!

35

Fall is a great time of year,
I never realized how great it was!

36

Funny the things you love
when you were never
exposed to them ...

37

The time is flying fast ...

2009

38

It has been quite a year.
I have many things to do ...

39

It is truly remarkable as to where I was
last August ...

40

Charlene has been and will always
mean and be everything to me ...

41

My personal legend ... to help others
and get people to the next level or
phase in their life

42

House is sold ... Good bye Amston ...
It was the best!

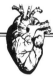

43

Looking at Banner

44

It has to be about Char and me now,
no one else ...

45

Sean back in the hospital ...

46

Char and I need to experience life
more than working and living ...

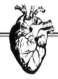

47

I think I found my calling –
it is to help others ...

48

Help people get to where they need
to be ... get them to the next level ...
help them be all that they can be ...

49

That's what we need to do ...
make each other feel special!

50

When I feel low I think of Sean ...
What am I complaining about?

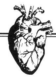

51

I will find a mentoring position ...

52

Wished I had written more ...

53

Sean has rejection ...

54

It feels good to work out!

55

I am still saying my prayers,
they seem to work well ...

56

My golf game was not bad ...
I just need to be more consistent ...

57

Declan is beautiful ...

58

Sean is on huge doses of prednisone ...

59

When we move into the condo
a chapter of the book is closed,
and another begins ...

60

I am ready to work with kids again ...

61

Sean still in hospital ... don't know
what lies ahead for him ...

62

It's all in God's hands!

63

What I do best is help others ...

64

Do whatever it takes ...

65

I have never felt so charged to establish
an idea or notion to help others ...

66

I know I did right
but then I start to doubt ...

67

I want to write that book ...

68

I am doing what is right and good ...

69

On You Tube ... imagine that!

70

I don't know how he does it …
He is positive and upbeat …

71

Sean has a prayer shawl and uses it!

72

We leave VA and head up to Boston ...
my, that is a lot of driving, but totally
worth it ...

73

I am fine ...

74

Speed up then, slowdown that ICD ...

75

Go back June of 2010 ...

76

Back to VA ...

77

All of us are in the room
for the doctor's words ...

78

Nothing else can be done for Sean ...
it's a matter of time!

79

Many choices must be made
when you are nearing death ...

80

Wow ... seems like it is not really
happening ...

81

Things will never be the same ...

82

Completely overwhelming ...

83

Sean says it's the last Christmas
because everybody is here ...

84

I feel devoid of emotion ... I don't know
what I want to do, say, or feel ....

85

Writings cannot capture the shot ...

86

Sometimes it seems like this is not happening and everything will go back to the way it was ...

2010

87

Haven't written much lately ...
can't seem to get my brain
around too much ...

88

I want to write a book,
but I can't seem to focus

89

I hear about these folks
who died of cardiac arrest due to an
enlarged heart, yet I did not ...

90

This is God's way of letting me know
that I have not accomplished all that I
am supposed to do ...

91

Now just push me
in the right direction ...

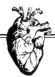

92

I know that I can truly
make a difference ...

93

Some type of schedule for my day
really helps ...

94

I need to call Sean tomorrow ...

95

My father died 38 years ago ...
seems like only yesterday ...

96

You know, when someone dies
you never really get over it ...
You learn how to live with it ...

97

Never give up and pursue your dreams

98

I am getting a second chance ...

99

Even if no one ever reads this,
or doesn't want to read this
I feel I have had an impact ...

100

How different my life has become ...

101

I am never satisfied ...
I am always restless ...

102

What do you say to someone
when they are losing their child?

103

It is a whole change of lifestyle
and making conscious choices
about what you consume ...

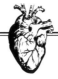

104

It's amazing the things you can
accomplish when you think you are
doing nothing ...

105

I figure that if I can control my diet,
exercise, and help others the rest
will fall into place ...

106

I have no idea what Sean goes through
day after day but if he is anything like
me, he has a strong desire to live ...

107

The little things we moan and groan about pale in comparison to the thoughts of a dying person ...

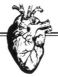

108

Ah yes, the quirky things we do ...

109

How is it when you get some money
and you swear you will save it,
you end up spending it on stuff ...

110

Sometimes I long for simpler times
when things weren't such a hassle ...

111

Nowadays it seems like we are on a
treadmill and living day to day ...

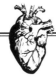

112

Lucky for me that I have dreams
and aspirations that keep me moving
in a good direction ...

113

It seems as all the governing powers
are corrupt and riddled with hypocrisy

114

Being gay and Catholic you are made
to believe that you will rot in hell,
but I know that is not true ...
I strive to live my life in a way
that I serve God, myself, and others ...

115

Nowadays it's real hard to find good
examples of what religion is all about ...

116

Maybe I will pray for all our
so-called religious leaders ...

117

Maybe tomorrow I will wake up and
this world will be a better place ...

118

2 years ago, I am laying in a hospital
bed ... Today I am riding on the train ...

119

Today is the tomorrow you worried
about yesterday ...

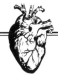

120

I did not want the view of the roof of
St. Francis Hospital to be my last one ...
yeeha it wasn't ...

121

It's the little things in life
that you come to enjoy such as walks
and other simple pleasures

122

As long as I have my dreams and
wishes, I feel alive and full of hope ...

123

You never know what is in store for someone ...

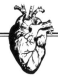

124

Maybe the best way for me to reach as many people as I can is to share the fact that everyone goes through things in their lives, but it is how we emerge from those experiences that determines the true value of life itself ...

125

When I begin to feel sorry for myself,
I am able to compensate by being
determined to help others and feeling
more and more energized on being
a part of something that is
bigger than me ...

126

Dreams ... this is how our loved ones
remain in our hearts and our minds ...

127

It is always helpful to have an objective,
empathetic, and non-judgmental
person to listen to your goings on ...

128

Funny how life can change in an
instant ...

129

The attitude that you take with you
on your life-changing path determines
what you will do when you land back
on solid ground ...

130

You can look back and be bitter about
what has happened to you or you can
see it as a new adventure ...

131

I prefer a new adventure ...

132

I want to give folks hope when they find themselves in situations that appear to be insurmountable ...

133

It is about others, not all about me ...
what a great place this would be if all
thought this way ...

134

It's amazing how you can use
your imagination to make things
seem real ...

135

We need to learn how to accept things
graciously and move on ...

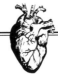

136

Looks like I am progressing a little ...

137

Sean not doing well ...

138

Life is supposed to get simpler as you
get older ... NOT

139

If anyone told me two years ago I would
be back to playing tennis, I never would
have believed them ...

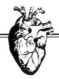

140

My health hasn't been the greatest
in the last two years, but I am
working at it ...

141

Attitude is everything ...

142

If I put my mind to something,
I can accomplish it ...

143

Everyone has a story to tell ...

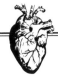

144

I always look up when I go outside ...

145

I always feel good after doing
something good for others ...

146

When I left the house, I looked up into
the big blue sky and I felt free again ...

147

We need to bring back respect and love
to one another ...

148

I get very tired, but it lets me know that
I am alive ...

149

I feel very deeply that all of us
need to be concerned more about
each other and do things that will
help lift all our spirits ...

150

No one seems to agree on helping those
who are less fortunate ... It's like some
of us want to leave them behind ....

151

This weighs heavy on my mind
and I pray for the world ...
come to think of it I pray a lot ...

152

Who realized that our thoughts
can be catalysts for change
and keeping ourselves headed
in a positive direction ...

153

Why do we have to be surrounded
by negativity ... ?

154

Can you imagine if everyone focused
on helping each other and taking care
of our world ... ? I wish ...

155

If changes need to be made,
it needs to begin with me ...

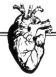

156

Age and illness are funny things ...
they make you reflect and spur you
into action ...

157

I have to do something
to keep my mind active ...

158

None of us know when our end
is coming so, live life to the fullest ...

159

Go Seanie ...

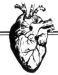

160

When we are having difficulties
with anything or when we are
emotional, make it a point
not to make comments ...

161

I have learned to listen to my body ...

162

Every day is a gift and an adventure ...

163

Goals are things that can sustain
anyone and everyone ...

164

All of us need to learn how
to take care of ourselves ...

165

Every day is a good day to be alive ...

166

From every happening and event
we learn a lesson ...

167

I wanted to call my mother ...

168

It's startling how you can
spend a whole day doing nothing ...
some days are like that ...

169

A new direction ...

170

I believe that with a conscious effort
you can be the things you need and
want to be ...

171

You start to look at your own life
and wonder what you have really
done with it ...

172

How many can say they have been
at death's door and now you are
out on the porch ...

173

Surround yourself with family
and friends who will always tell you
like it is, like it or not ...

174

You can learn a lot
by observing a person ...

175

Sean ... no complaints, excuses,
or poor me ...

176

Life is great, life is a journey ...
just when you think you are
at the end of your trip, you head down
another path ...

177

I am not going to give up ...

178

I am trying very hard to remain
positive about all the things
going on in my life ...

179

There isn't a day that I don't think at one time or another, about my heart ...

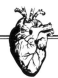

180

It's amazing how much time you can waste on a computer ...

181

I hope that when I move on to the next life that people will look at me as someone who aspired to be the best she could be for herself and for others ...

182

I was longing for a simpler time ...

183

It's good to have goals ...
it helps and guides us ...
and makes all things possible ....

184

Cherish your life people, you don't
know how good you have it ...

185

Look after me Lord and help me do
what I am supposed to do ...

186

We talked about death, Darby, Gram,
and his decision to donate his organs to
medical research and/or transplant ...
It was his way of giving back ...

187

When you die it is your spirit
that is most important ...

188

You can't go backwards ...

189

The doctor was right ... there is no way
I could keep the schedule I had before
March 17, 2008 ...

190

Tomorrow is a new day ...

191

Why is it that some folks can go
through life without any real obstacles
and then there are some of us who have
to deal with obstacles as a matter of
living ...

192

Somewhere it is written that God never
gives us more than we can handle,
but did he/she have to give some folks
so much ...

193

It takes thirty seconds for an emotion
to run through your brain, but it is up
to us to decide whether to keep it going
or end it ...

194

All of us have some form of spirituality
to help guide us through life ...

195

You lose yourself when you devote
yourself to others ...

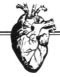

196

I am keeping on with my positive
thoughts hoping that my synergy will
align with the universe and get all of us
headed in the right direction ...

197

Sat outside tonight and enjoyed it ...
I miss the simple things ...

198

How far I have come
and how far I have yet to go ...

199

I called my mother's phone today ...
I feel better when I am finished
calling her ...

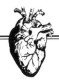

200

It is in your perspective ...

201

I need to start feeling settled,
but it is hard for me ...

202

There is nothing like rearranging your
space to give yourself a boost ...

203

It's funny when you don't have something to do, you wish you had something to do and when you wish you had nothing to do, you have something to do ...

204

Melancholy came over me tonight ... The secret is pushing through and thinking about how you have been blessed by many things ...

205

He struggles with his illness ...

206

It is a miracle that I have my own heart
and am able to be a bit physical ...

207

I feel like I am sinking a bit ...

208

After a scream of I hate our life this morning, I took a ride in the car, got my act together, went to get blood drawn, got a coffee and changed my whole disposition ...

209

Why do things have to be so difficult ...

210

Sean is 34 ...

211

Mish mash of emotions ... ups and
downs and nothings ... every day seems
to be a drag ...

212

I need to get on my upside ...

213

One day you look at yourself and you
look pretty good, the next day you look,
and it seems you aged 5 years ...

214

Dr. appointment ... good news my heart
is still beating, and I continue on a
good path ...

215

I need to continue on me ...
a work in progress ...

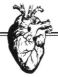

216

There is beauty to be found
everywhere ...

217

Couldn't sleep ... Feels like there is a lot
on my mind but of no consequences ...

218

Why is it so much easier for me to write
things other than say them out loud ...?

219

When you worry it is usually about something from the past or in the future ...

220

I really cannot afford to not take care of myself ...

221

It's tough moving backwards
but the good part is that it means
you have a lot of room to manipulate in
and improve upon ...

222

I am fighting really hard to come to
grips with the way I feel at times ...

223

Everything feels hard to do right now ...

224

I need to live in the present, but I want
the future to be the present ...

225

I think some prayers are being
answered ...

226

A little worried about myself
and I need your help ...

227

I constantly self-talk ...
all in a good way ...
you have to do that ...
be mindful of what you say and do ...

228

I don't know about you, but I am always
looking for ways to improve and make
the present and future bright ...

229

I am thankful for everything ...

230

Sometimes you just have to pull
yourself up by the bootstraps
and move on ...

231

No one can ever give us
a clear date on our departure ...

232

I wrote down my goals
and keep them with me ...

233

I gave my all to whatever I did
and was able to accomplish much ...

234

Lots of dreams going on ...

235

Maybe we are not supposed
to think about it ... just live ...

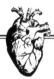

236

Sean looking thin and frail ...
mom all over again ...

2011

237

A new year and new energy ...

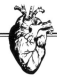

238

I am like hardwood floors ... you tear
up the carpets and you realize what you
have been walking on, all along ...

239

It is not what you were then
but what you are now ...

240

Love looking at those stars ...

241

There is a lot going on
inside this head of mine ...

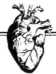

242

You deserve more ...

243

All good things come together,
sooner or later ...

244

It's all up to us to make this world
a better place ...

245

Thoughts center on helping others,
which in turn helps me ...

246

Do not neglect yourself
or your health ...

247

There is a special place in heaven
for the disabled ...

248

I feel I am waiting for a big change ...

249

You have it all (at least you think) and
then in an instant, all is different ...

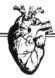

250

I feel sometimes that it is my fault that
all of this stuff is happening and then I
have to remind myself that everything
happens for a reason, and there is a
reason I am alive ...

251

I get my moments and then I try
to fill my head with all the positives
that have happened ...

252

Positives do outweigh the negatives ...

253

Not myself, just an overall feeling ...

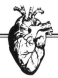

254

A curtain has come down
and it obscures my thoughts ...

255

I called her, she always responds ...

256

Calling all angels ...

257

All I can do is listen and be attentive ...
sometimes that is all we can do ...

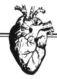

258

My writing imitates the communication
of today ... short, no real punctuation,
and misspelled ...

259

I believe that I am in a league of my
own ... always lived my life that way ...

260

Things seem to be closing in ...

261

I didn't realize that I had so many
dreams ...

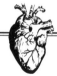

262

Maybe I am only meant
to be a dreamer ...

263

Sometimes you want to be
somewhere different ...

264

Do things always have to be
so difficult ...

265

I realize no pain, no gain but
every once in a while, it would be nice
to have a reprieve ...

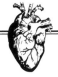

266

Was off course but now back on track ...

267

I want a nice smooth sail ...
Is that too much to ask ...

268

There has to be more to life
than just here ...

269

I believe that many people are going
through these same struggles ...

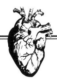

270

Lift yourself out of the barrel ...

271

His story needs to be told ...

272

Lots of stuff going on ...

273

I am ready for the sun
to shine upon my face ...

274

It seems as if my body is trying
to tell me something ...

275

I still use my imagination today ...
thank God I have one ...

276

What if I write for years about
my thoughts, dreams, and aspirations
and no one cares ...

277

Then again, this stuff should matter the most to me and no one else ...

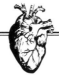

278

There is a lot to do
and I hope I can do all of it ...

279

He says he is feeling sad, and
here I am wanting to complain ....

280

Better days, maybe for me
but what about everyone else ...

281

I thought that life would get easier
as you got older, but I see it is filled
with a whole different set of issues ...

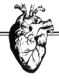

282

I have written 57,062 words ...

283

Why it so difficult for people to provide
good service to folks ...

284

If you are responsible for something
or some place, man up and do it ...

285

We struggle, and they live
free and easy ...

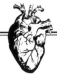

286

I sometimes write an edited version
of what I am thinking ...

287

I am always looking on the bright side
of things but there are days when I
question everything ...

288

On those dark days,
I fight my way through ...

289

Am I really helping others ...

290

Am I really making a difference ...

291

Am I doomed to live
only chasing dreams ... ?

292

Will I ever get ahead ... ?

293

Will my circumstances change ...

294

Is there something
I should be doing ... ?

295

What is it that I really want ...

296

I have so many questions some days,
it boggles my mind ...

297

There are some days I feel defeated ...

298

It is a constant battle, but the nice thing
is I can usually get myself back in the
right frame of mind ...

299

Every day is starting to feel the same ...

300

Tomorrow will come and I will put on
my mantle of everything is going to be
great ...

301

I feel I am having a hard time
focusing ...

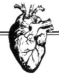

302

Today was the "I feel a little useless"
day ...

303

You should not tie up your identity
with your job ...

304

I always let on that everything is great
but, you know what? Sometimes they
are not ...

305

I do not like to perseverate
on the so-called bad day I am having ...

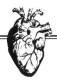

306

Tomorrow all these thoughts
will be reversed ...

307

Boy, am I in the zone ...

308

I really thought about nothing today ...
hard to believe, I know ...

309

Valentine's Day ... I never saw the
significance of this day ...

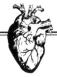

310

If you love someone, every day should
be Valentine's Day ...

311

Had a breakfast at the HS
with Rotary, I do miss being at school
with kids and staff ...

312

It is always good to have someone
who knows your pain ...

313

The day goes by fast ...
It is disconcerting sometimes ...

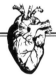

314

Dr. Carelink ...
technology is amazing ...

315

What would happen
if all this technology and meds
were not in the equation ...

316

In the old days, I would be dead ...

317

I have no idea how he remains ... If the
will is strong, the body will follow ...

318

How long can someone continue
in this state ...

319

It is way beyond my scope of knowing
things ...

320

I have so many self-doubts ...

321

I don't feel like doing anything ...

322

I am feeling that this is all there will
ever be and that is not good ...

323

I am feeling a bit depressed and am
trying to keep my spirits up by telling
myself that I am only one step away
from breaking things open for me ...

324

Sometimes I want to scream why is all
this crap happening to me ...

325

You have to deal with what you have ...

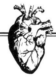

326

My life right now is the biggest
challenge I have had so far ...

327

I moved myself into a good position,
in terms of positive thinking ...

328

Sean has pneumonia ...
what else could happen to this kid ...

329

It does not seem fair ...

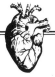

330

Life sure comes at you fast
and with a vengeance ...

331

It is great to be involved in your area ...

332

It is like reinventing me ...

333

I am doing some reading which is
making me rethink all that I am ...

334

I like having thoughts in my head
to focus me ...

335

I hope everyone can experience
the feeling of making a difference ...

336

There is a special place in heaven
for all those who have had to fight
their way through life with an unfair
advantage and an inability to take care
of themselves ...

337

I want to be known as the one who
tried to help ...

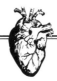

338

It is frustrating to have no control over
what is happening and not having a
real way of doing anything other than
listen and be supportive ...

339

I can't quite figure out what lesson in
life is to be learned here ...

340

You never know what you are going to
get an any given day, so you might as
well roll with the punches ...

341

There is so much feeling and emotion
here that it is nearly impossible to
relate what is going on ...

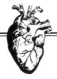

342

I had a conversation
with mom in the car ...

343

Though I write many thoughts down
here, there are far more that go through
my head all day ...

344

I am really filled with a lot of questions
to myself ...

345

I repeat myself at times ...

346

Looked in the mirror ...
boy have I aged ...

347

You age in 5-year increments ...

348

The CD for Sean is almost done ...

349

You have to have some goal
to believe in ...

350

If you want to help people
there are some out there who would
say that these folks need to fend for
themselves or their families need to
take care of them ...

351

Stay the course Kate,
you are doing the right thing ....

352

He sleeps a lot now and is very weak ...

353

You feel good doing things for others ...

354

My mind is too active to shut off ...

355

I need to do better at shutting off
internal noises ...

356

I am 100% responsible
for what happens ...

357

3 years ago ... dire straits ...

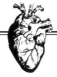

358

Thank god I am still here
to return favors ...

359

I want to do so much ...
I hope I can ...

360

Not in the mood to think
or anything else ...

361

Social action is such a great thing ...

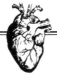

362

I think I can live anywhere ...

363

I need to be sure that I am not
overdoing it ...

364

I need to walk more ...

365

I believe in the power
of positive thinking ...

366

I am looking for a little more solitude ...

367

Family is important ...

368

No thinking ... just relax ...

369

Let's see what tomorrow brings ...

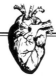

370

Positive and happy ...
See it, feel it, live it, read it ...

371

Sluggish but got some things done ...

372

Then I will take time to be grateful
for the things that were good today ...

373

Sean weak ...

374

Pray for them all ... you really don't
know what else to do and then again
maybe this is all you can do ...

375

A real test of faith ...

376

I am not in the mood to do much,
but I push myself ...

377

Why is it that some float through life
without a scratch ... ?

378

It seems all things will work out ...

379

Dinner with friends is always nice ...

380

There is always tomorrow ...

381

I can do anything
if I set my mind to it ...

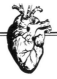

382

Could not get settled
with things today ...

383

I am emoted out ...

384

As long as I am trying my best,
that's what matters ...

385

Live in the present ...

386

Do what you do
and when you don't feel right, stop ...

387

I want a miracle
where everything is great ...

388

Told him I loved him and don't be
afraid ...

389

Sean died ... He was 34 years old and
an incredibly strong willed and great
person ...

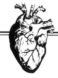

390

Very overwhelming ...

2012

391

Another year, another chance
to do good ...

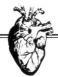

392

Help all to be the very best
they can be ...

393

Start all over again ...

394

What you give comes back to you ...

395

The universe is mine ... connect to it!

396

I won't be deterred!

397

Faith is more than a preacher
in church ...

398

Obviously, nun = none to them ...
Wake up Padre!

399

Unsettled and looking for calm ...

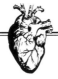

400

If nothing else, thinking of all the things you are grateful for, really changes your perspective ...

401

Take my body Jesus ...

402

Good Morning, world!

403

Mom it's your 6th anniversary, what are
your and Sean's conversations like?

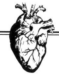

404

Gratitude does work, and I saw it in
action today ...

405

Not everyone is perfect,
and neither am I ...

406

It's harder than you think,
to start a revolution ...

407

Look for signs everywhere ...

408

Pray and choose to be positive

409

Never underestimate
the power of prayer ...

410

For a split second, doubt ...
then wonder and awe ...

411

You choose your own mood
so choose wisely ...

412

Reintroduce myself to low sodium ...

413

Maybe I should blog again ...

414

There but for the grace of God, go I ...

415

It is what it is ...

416

Start little by little ... It's okay!

417

How could I forget Theresa?

418

It's a small world and getting smaller ...

419

Rewind ... Start all over
but do it better ...

420

Will this be the day?
I hope ... Get busy Kate!

421

Don't start the day off all revved up
by the wrong reasons ...

422

Come back to the center ...
That's where you belong ...

423

Today is going to be a great day!

424

Look for all the little surprises!

425

Everything is here for you to use ...

426

Use things wisely!

427

Be the best you can be!

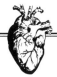

428

Follow a life routine, a ritual ... It's comforting, uplifting. And hopeful ...

429

Too much information
is not a good thing ...

430

Live life as it comes ...

431

Take care of today!

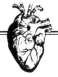

432

Find what you like and go from there ...

433

My thoughts have been scattered
but I am trying to refocus ... Writing,
meditation will help, prayer too!

434

I am counting on them all ...

435

Waiting, but enjoying ...

436

Thoughts and prayers with everyone
for the next couple of hours, days, and
forever! See you all on the flip side ...

437

Prayers for those who have lost much ...

438

God rest your soul Ray! You were good
to us and Darby ...

439

Until we meet again ...

440

I gotta get back to when I was
self-aware and taking better
care of myself ...

441

The power of positive thinking is
endless ...

442

People making demands ...
Yes, I will quiet down ...
Just don't judge anyone ...

443

With you and me, I can do anything!

444

A never-ending battle to resist the negative and keep it from spiraling, but ... I can do anything!

445

Have more than I started with today ...
and more all of my life ...

446

Happy for some and sad for others and
then it starts all over again ...

447

The first snow can be a sign of
things to come ...

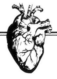

448

I am thinking positive thoughts ...
I am positive the sun will come out
and melt all the snow away ...
No shoveling for you!

449

Start off slow and moody, work my way
out of it, pray, and be grateful for what I
have ... and I have much in comparison
to others ...

450

Be grateful ...

451

Maybe I have cheated a bit, but I can restart today trying to do my best ...

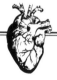

452

Do not over extend yourself ... Sometimes I need to think of me in a health perspective ...

453

Start the holiday season
by being grateful ...

454

Accomplish what you set out to do in
the morning and you will feel renewed,
invigorated, and at peace
with yourself ...

455

It's better, thank you very much ...

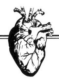

456

The weeks get better and better
as they go along ...

457

How great it is to give to others!

458

Something wonderful
will happen today, no matter
how big or how small ...

459

Follow your premonitions ...
they have a point of truth ...

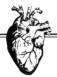

460

Feel better already!

461

December 14, 2012 ...
gone but not to be forgotten!

2013

462

You always want what you don't have
but is that any way to live?

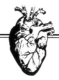

463

Every day find new ways and new ideas
to be thankful that you are alive ...

464

Pray for others, it helps you overcome
the negative thoughts!

465

Something wonderful will happen
today and every day ...

466

Negative thoughts spiral and before
you know it you are lost in them ...
Stop and go back! Positive spirals
are much better ...

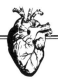

467

Always come up with things
to be thankful for ...

468

It's when you stop being thankful that
your world will come to an end ...

469

Do things before it is too late ...

470

Enjoy now because you will
be busy later!

471

Where can I make the biggest
difference?

472

Rest your soul Bill and enjoy the
presence of the Lord and all your
family that has gone before you ...

473

The start ... now if I can only see it
through to the finish ...

474

Better focus ... Did I ever really have it?

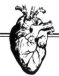

475

Your own is better than anything else!

476

I need to chronicle my journey ...
it will help me and help others ...

477

Inspiration, passion, and
perseverance ... come back ...
I need you, I want you, and
give me the spark ...

478

Anticipate great things happening
and they will!

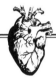

479

Prepare for success

480

Got married!

481

Take the spotlight off yourself ...
others need your help as well ...
Libby, Dennis, and Hart need you!

482

I am ready to serve ...

483

Don't wait ... just do it!

484

Now is the time to do it!

485

Accepted into the transplant
program ... hard to believe!

486

Now is the time I need to shut down
some things and take better care of
myself and others ...

487

I must be more patient
and accepting of myself!

488

Help me stay strong!

489

I am still here ... there is a reason
and I will find it!

490

Bring on the new heart!

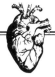

491

Every day wake up
and give thanks to all!

492

Motivation to write please!
Motivation to exercise please!
I am a little short on it ...

493

If pain doesn't go away I should call ...
Help it go away!

494

Keep moving forward!

495

You can get upset but what you do after
the upset is most important ...

496

Maybe I ought to do a few more walks
with less time ...

497

I can feel my strength coming back ...

498

Focus is an issue, but it will get better ...

499

Write things day by day ... they are
much easier to remember ...

500

One can only hope and pray!

501

Thank you for everything
you have given me!

502

Look on the bright side of things ...
there is no time for darkness ...

503

Keep pushing through ...

504

Thinking about and helping others
is speeding up my recovery ...

505

Think of others!

506

Keep moving forward and have faith ...

507

I want Dennis to be healed
and I want a new heart ...

508

Something magical will happen,
believe it!

509

Humility and a positive attitude are
what you need ...

510

You get what you give so remain
positive, loving, and caring ...

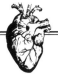

511

Have positive thinking,
be non-judgmental, and stay away
from negative conversations
and influences ...

512

Avoid the pitfalls of being upset or
bothered by things and then taking
them out on the ones you love ...

513

No one knows what direction or course
your life will take, so live life to the
fullest and love to the fullest ...

514

I will continue to have faith and pray for Dennis's recovery ... I know you can heal him, Lord ... and all the angels and saints ...

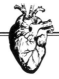

515

Life is a gift! Open it, live it, love it, and thank God for it!

516

Your will be done ...

517

It's times like these that really test your faith and beliefs but without them you would have nothing!

518

October 30th, Dennis dies ... Bring his
soul to heaven! I love you and will miss
you! You and Sean are together!

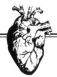

519

You will never be forgotten ...

520

Family is important!

521

Mom, Dad, Sean and Dennis are
celebrating mom's birthday ... Enjoy!

522

Judy – 60th birthday ...
Wow, time passes extremely fast ...
Where does it go!

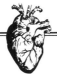

523

Gratitude and happiness are two
important things in my life ...

524

Be thankful and happy
and all falls into place ...

525

I believe strongly that if you continue to
compliment, encourage, and tell others
the great things that they can become,
you can also do that for yourself ...

526

Make others worthy, because they are worthy ... The same is true for yourself ...

527

Thank you, Thank you, Thank you!

528

Living your life and gratitude …

529

It is difficult to be non-judgmental
and thankful … We all need to remind
ourselves to do these things …

530

We are all warriors fighting a battle
against the negative ideas that infiltrate
our thinking and lives each day ... We
can be successful if we keep at it and
live what it is we seek!

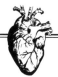

531

Do what you like ... like what you do!

532

Become your dreams!

533

You are capable of everything!

534

Shut up and listen!

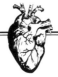

535

Searching for the divine means
changes of actions, thoughts, and
words ...

536

I am ... I can ...

537

Seek and ye shall find ...

538

I may not be rich, but I am alive,
wealthy, grateful, and happy ...

539

I lost a day to illness, but it is okay ...
I am starting to come back ...

540

What you are and what you manifest
can be one and the same ...

541

I am that I am ...

542

Do not settle for anything less unto
which you aspire ...

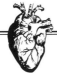

543

The best present – my presence ...

544

Let it come to me ...
sit down, shut up, and listen ...

545

How wonderful to be
surrounded by friends ...

546

I lost a year but gained a life ...

2014

547

Starting over is great!

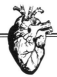

548

Begin anew and hold fast!

549

Let no one take
these dreams from you ...

550

You are the master of your
hopes and dreams ...

551

If no one should ever see or read
these words, what will it matter?
It has made all the difference for me!

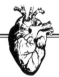

552

You really don't know how strong
you are until the situation arises
and you muster that strength ...

553

Death is random ...

554

Your own issues make you look at your
own mortality ...

555

You can never be too grateful for the things you have and the things you have been given ...

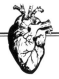

556

I will carry on with the will and strength of a warrior, keeping myself focused on the good in myself and the good in others ...

557

When you stop learning,
you stop living.

558

I am happy, I am healthy, I am holy,
I am wealthy, I am loving, I am caring,
I am strong, and I am harmonious

559

I am light, I am love, I am peace,
and I am joy ...

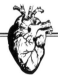

560

The I ams have it ...

561

Let peace begin with me ...

562

When you want to write down thoughts, how come you can't find them?

563

Nothing is ever lost.
It's merely misplaced ...

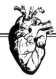

564

If you want to admire me, that's okay.
I am only doing the best I can ...

565

It takes a lot of work to be an
inspirational thinker ...

566

You can serve others through your
words and thoughts ...

567

Often, I wish to see for one more time,
the faces of whom I have lost ...

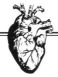

568

I will always find ways to lift my
spirit ... being melancholic is not for
me ...

SEPTEMBER 26, 2014

I got the call – My heart is in ...

SEPTEMBER 27, 2014

Heart Transplant — Brigham and Women's Hospital

And so, a new life begins ...
And so, a new chapter begins ...

Unbelievable and Forever Grateful!

A Chronology of Medical Events

2008

- March 2008 – Visit to the Emergency Medical Center
- Transported to hospital, hospitalized
- Diagnosis of heart failure
- Life Vest or external defibrillator worn home
- Medication
- Blood Draws
- Visit to Cardiologist CT
- April 2008 – I want a second opinion
- MA - Brigham And Women's Hospital
- Diagnosis confirmed.
- Ditch the Life Vest or External defibrillator
- Placement of an ICD (Implanted Cardiac Defibrillator) – Brigham and Women's Hospital
- Medication, medication change
- Blood Draws
- Visits to the cardiologist CT and MA – Brigham and Women's Hospital

2009

- Medication
- Medication changes
- Blood Draws
- Cardiologist visits CT and MA - Brigham and Women's Hospital

2010

- Medication
- Medication changes
- Blood Draws
- Cardiologist visits CT and MA - Brigham and Women's Hospital

2011

- Medication
- Medication changes
- Blood Draws
- Cardiologist visits CT and MA - Brigham and Women's Hospital

2012

- Medication
- Medication changes
- Blood Draws
- Cardiologist visits CT and MA - Brigham and Women's Hospital

2013

- Medication
- Medication changes
- Blood Draws
- Cardiologist visits MA - Brigham and Women's Hospital
- Severe heart failure
- Gall Bladder Surgery
- Hospitalizations – Brigham and Women's Hospital
- Transplant Evaluation – Brigham and Women's Hospital
- Accepted into the Transplant Program at Brigham and Women's Hospital
- Implantation of the Left Ventricular Assist Device (LVAD – internal heart pump) – Brigham and Women's Hospital
- Placement on the Transplant List

2014

- Medication
- Cardiologist visits MA – Brigham and Women's Hospital
- LVAD Clinic Visits MA – Brigham and Women's Hospital
- Blood Draws
- Replace ICD
- Phone call – My heart is in – September 26, 2014
- Heart Transplant – September 27, 2014 at Brigham and Women's Hospital

A Chronology of Personal Events

2008
- School Principal
- Diagnosis Heart Failure
- Hospitalization
- Possible heart transplant
- Give up my Principalship
- Change my diet ... low sodium
- Disability from Teacher Retirement
- Loss of 70% of income
- Put home on the real estate market
- Synergy Center is founded
- Start exercising, walking

2009
- Exercising, walking
- Continue with change of diet
- Home on the market
- Sale of Home
- Move to a rental home
- Co-founded a non-profit - Sensations Charitable Foundation, Inc
- Declan born

2010
- Exercising, walking, gym
- Sean in hospital
- Visits to Virginia
- Buy a condo
- Florida
- Outer Banks (Sean's last stay)
- Synergy and Sensations Charitable Foundation, Inc programs
- Running Social Skills Programs for Children
- East Haddam Rotary Member

2011

- Exercising, walking, gym
- Synergy and Sensations Charitable Foundation, Inc
- Social Skills Programs for Children
- Colchester Cares
- East Haddam Rotary Member
- Visits to Virginia
- Florida
- Sean dies, Memorial Service

2012

- Exercising, walking, gym
- Florida
- Colchester Cares
- Mentor student
- Synergy Center
- Sensations Charitable Foundation, Inc
- Social Skills Programs for Children
- Board Member - Special Education Program in Groton, CT
- East Haddam Rotary Member

2013

- Exercising, walking, gym
- Married Charlene
- Minis on the Dragon
- Colchester Cares
- Mentor student
- Synergy Center
- Sensations Charitable Foundation, Inc
- Social Skills Programs for Children
- Board Member – Special Education Program in Groton, CT
- East Haddam Rotary Member
- Dennis Jr. dies, Memorial Service

2014

- Exercising, walking, gym
- Florida
- Minis take the States – Buffalo to Bethlehem, PA route
- A new Mini
- Outer Banks
- Heart Transplant
- Synergy Center
- Sensations Charitable Foundation, Inc
- Social Skills Programs for Children
- Board Member – Special Education Program in Groton, CT
- Colchester Cares
- Mentor student
- East Haddam Rotary Member

KATE O'BOYLE

Kate is a life-long educator. Her 30+ years of career experiences have focused on helping children, their families, and the community at large. She served as a teacher, coach, mentor, guidance counselor, assistant principal, and a principal in the PA, MD, RI, and CT public schools. Upon being diagnosed with a serious 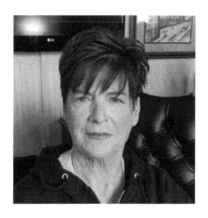 heart condition, she had to reinvent herself and use her skills in other ways to continue helping others.

Born and raised in Bethlehem, PA, she currently spends her time in Florida and Connecticut with her spouse.